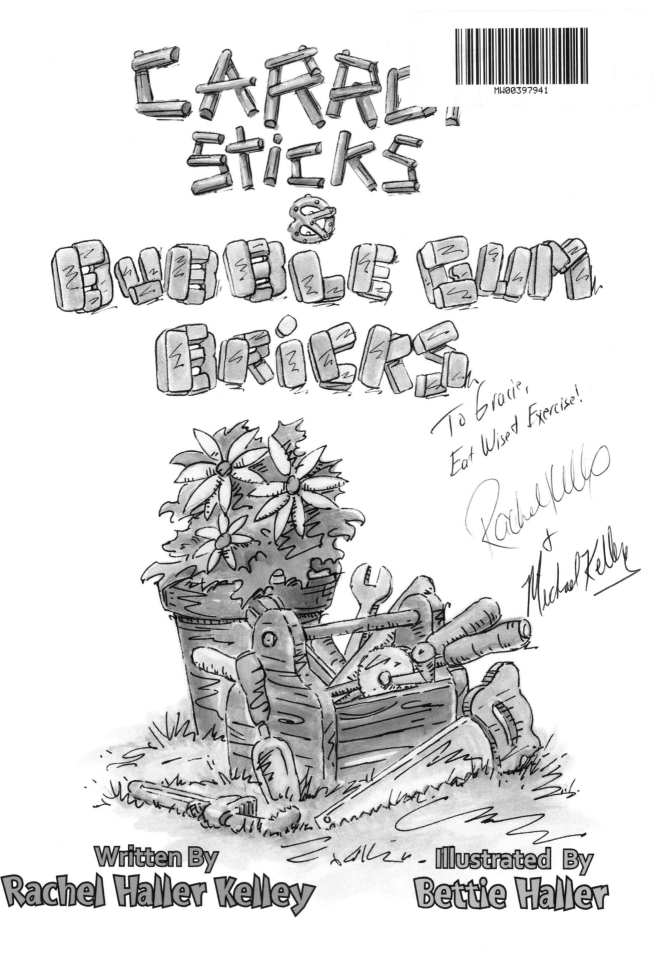

CARROT STICKS & BUBBLE GUM BRICKS

To Gracie,
Eat Wise & Exercise!

Rachel Kelley
&
Michael Kelley

Written By
Rachel Haller Kelley

Illustrated By
Bettie Haller

*This book is dedicated
to my husband, Michael,
who has encouraged and supported me
all along the way!
I love you!*

Christian Books and Games
P.O. Box 99
Pulaski, Tennessee 38478
www.ChristianBooksandGames.com

The text of this book is set in ITC Benguiat Book.
The illustrations are rendered in acrylic paint and ink.

Carrot Sticks & Bubble Gum Bricks/ by Rachel Haller Kelley;
Illustrated by Bettie Haller
Summary: Mama Eaton informs her two sons
that it's time to move out and make their own way in life.
Big Brother Eaton chooses to build his house out of healthy foods,
but Little Brother decides that sweets and greasy foods
are the way to go. But when a whirlwind of germs blows in and attacks their dwellings,
Big Brother's house stands firm,
but Little Brother's junk food house caves in, showing him
he was wrong, and that healthy foods make the best homes.
ISBN: 978-1481272261

Special thanks to Barbara Temple Davis
for her assistance in the editing of this book.

The Eaton brothers, playful and spry,
have gotten big so fast.
Their childhood was filled with laughter and thrills,
But now they're grown at last.

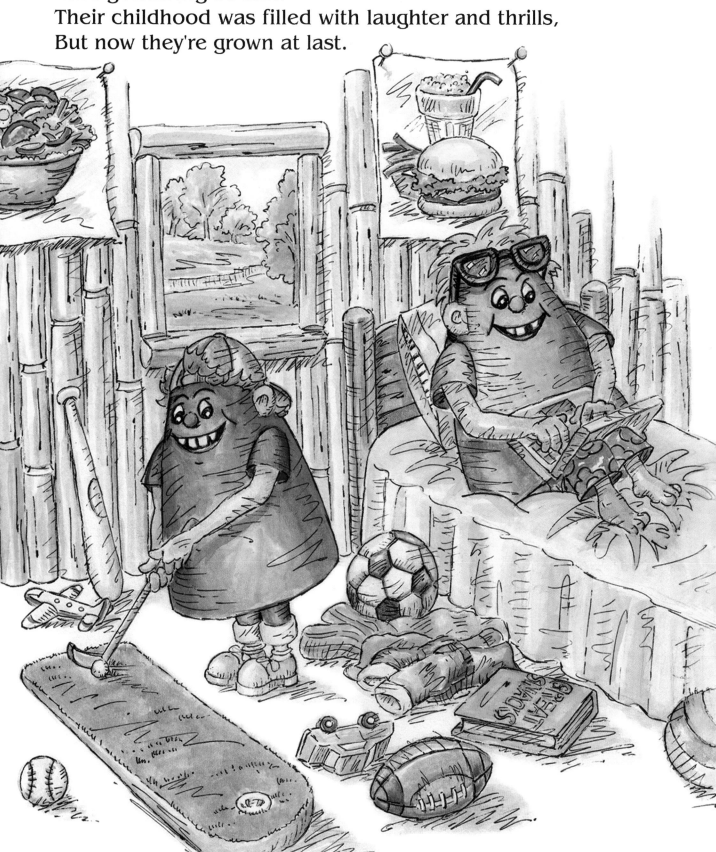

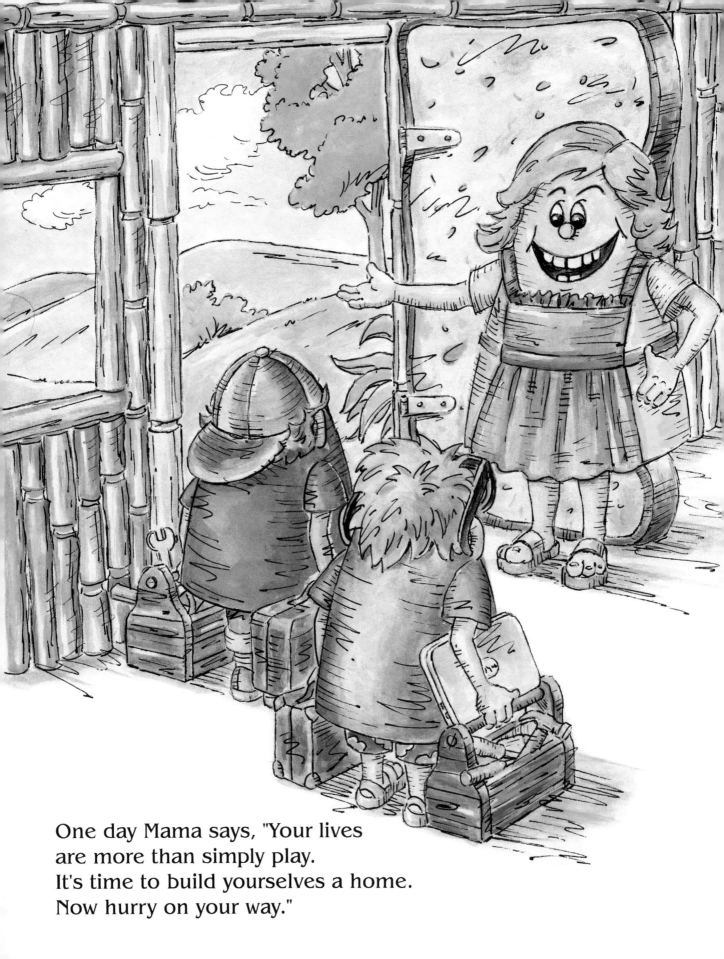

One day Mama says, "Your lives
are more than simply play.
It's time to build yourselves a home.
Now hurry on your way."

With luggage and tools, they leave their mom, excited to roam the hills.
"Where should we live?" they ask themselves.
"What kind of homes should we build?"

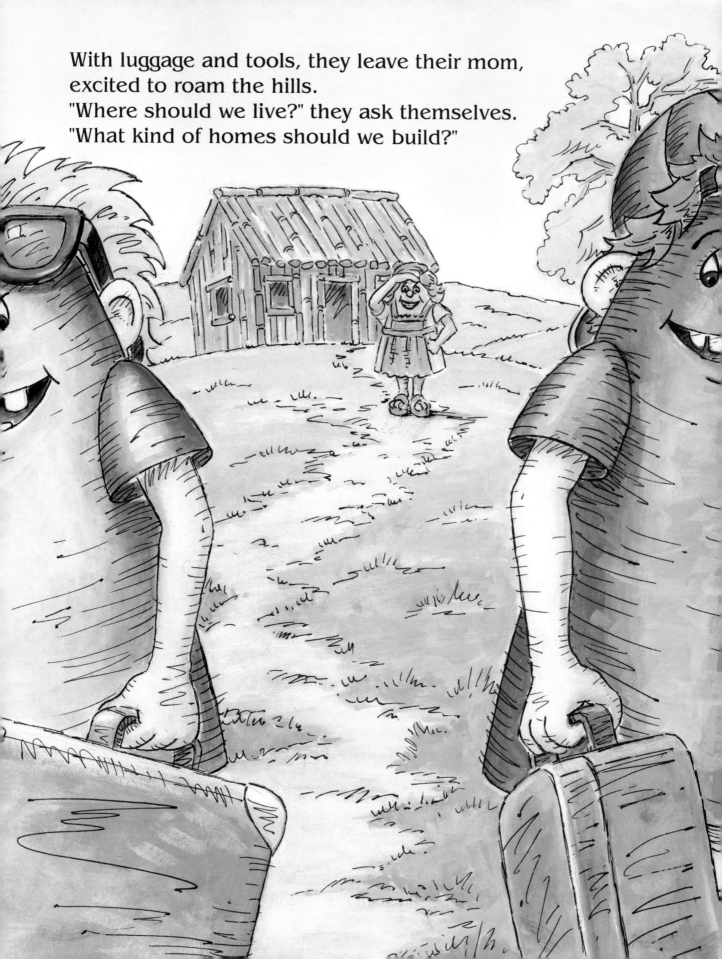

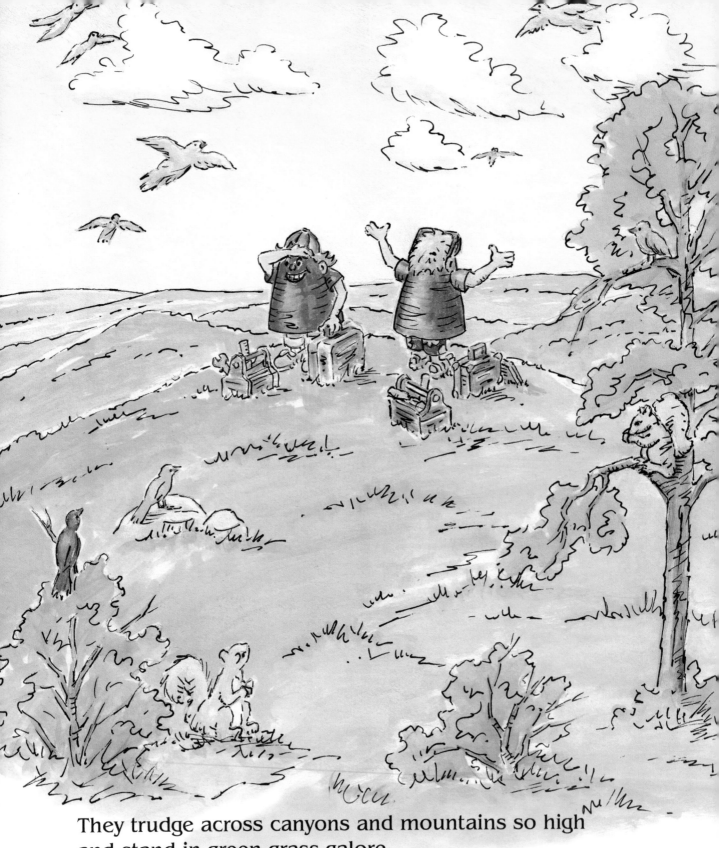

They trudge across canyons and mountains so high
and stand in green grass galore.
"Should we choose pastures or valleys?" they ask.
"What fun! Let's go and explore!"

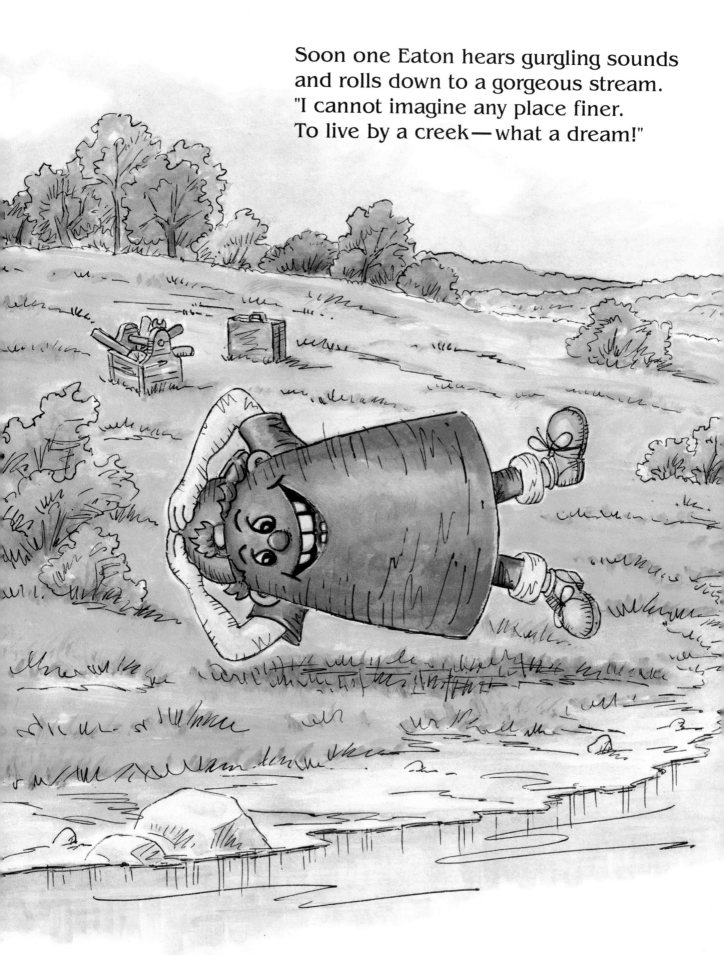

Soon one Eaton hears gurgling sounds
and rolls down to a gorgeous stream.
"I cannot imagine any place finer.
To live by a creek—what a dream!"

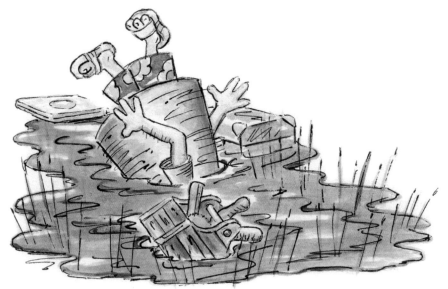

The other is drawn toward a muddy pond
and dives into the bog.

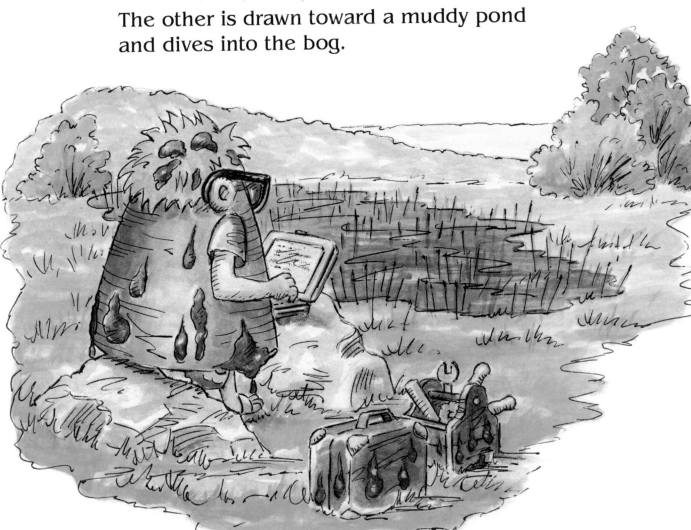

"It's perfect!" he says. "Just what I want.
I'll write it on my blog."

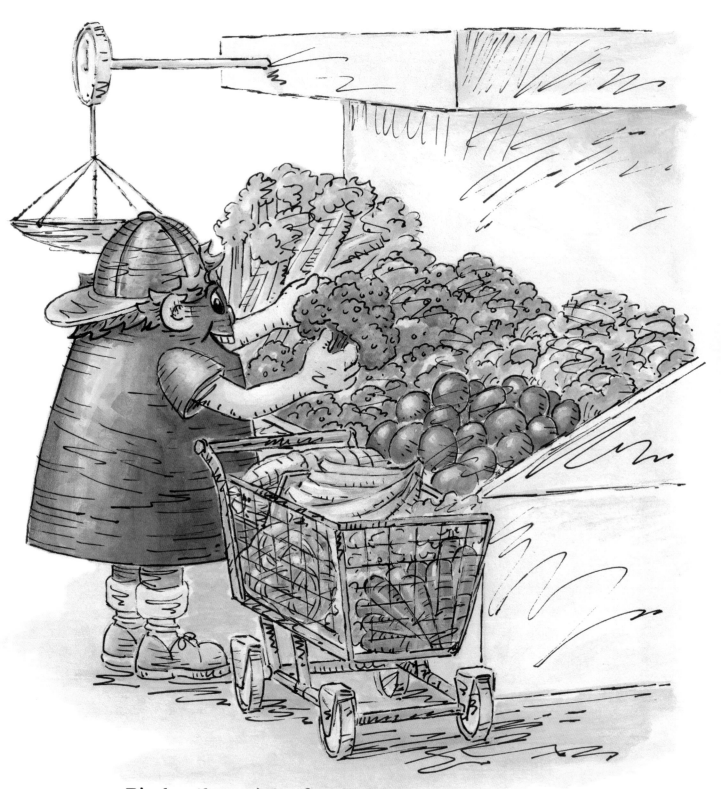

Big brother picks foods that are tasty and sturdy
to build a home solid and strong.
"Broccoli, celery, carrots, and beans—
smart choices will make it last long."

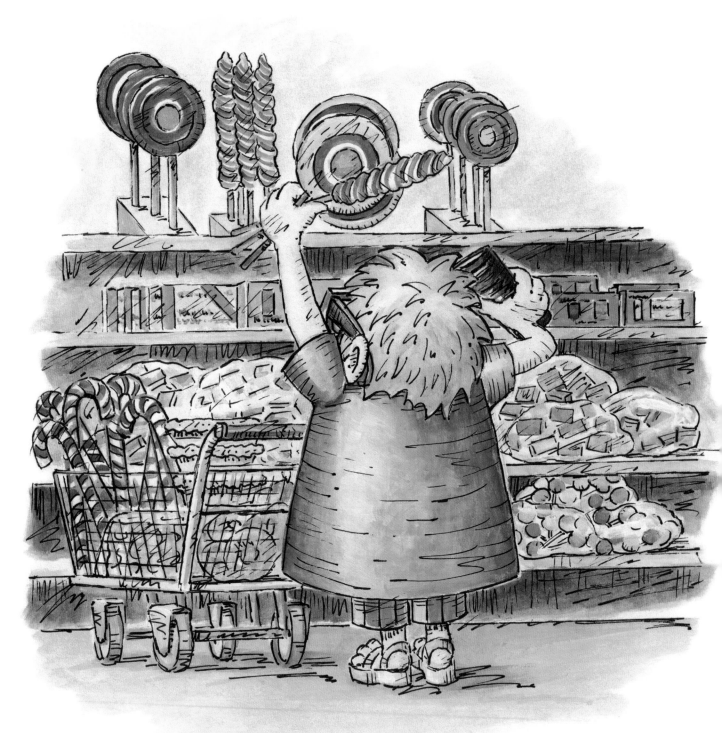

Little brother runs to the candy aisle
to load up on sugary treats.
"Suckers and gooey chocolates!
Anything goes if it's sweet."

"Green beans make my walls stand firm.
Carrot sticks strengthen the roof.
What can I use to bind them together?
Nut butter works. Here's the proof!"

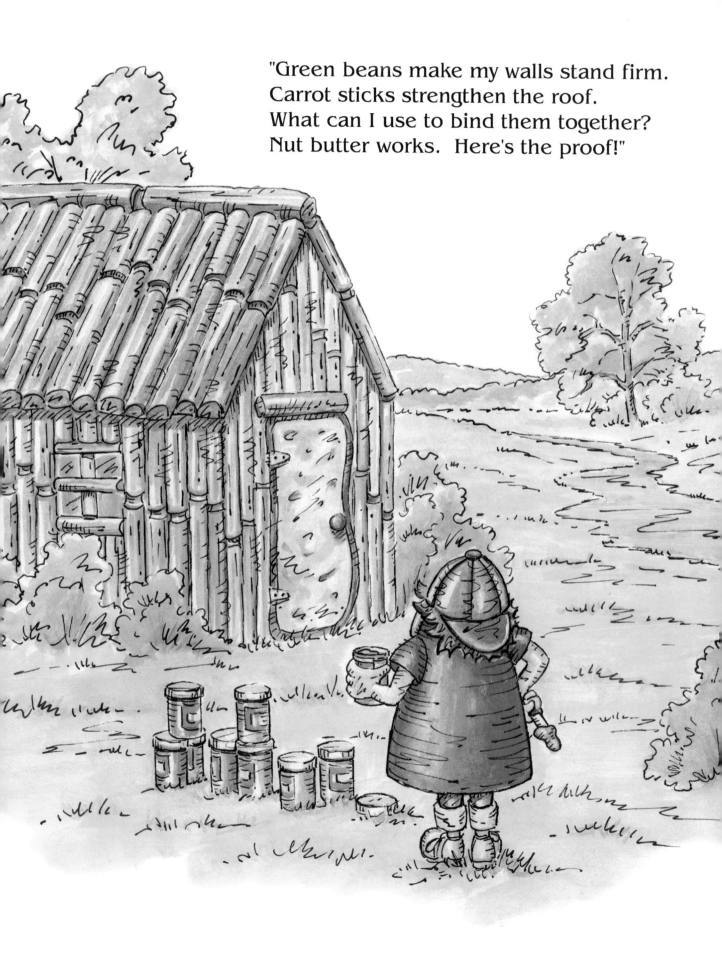

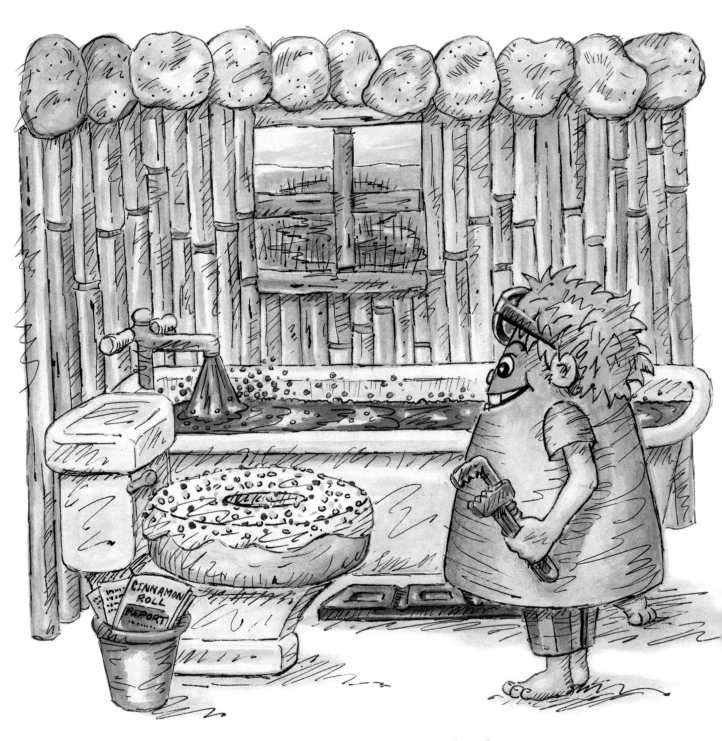

"Greasy fries give a tasty look.
Potato chips make it complete.
Can't wait to soak in a tub full of soda
and sit on my round doughnut seat!"

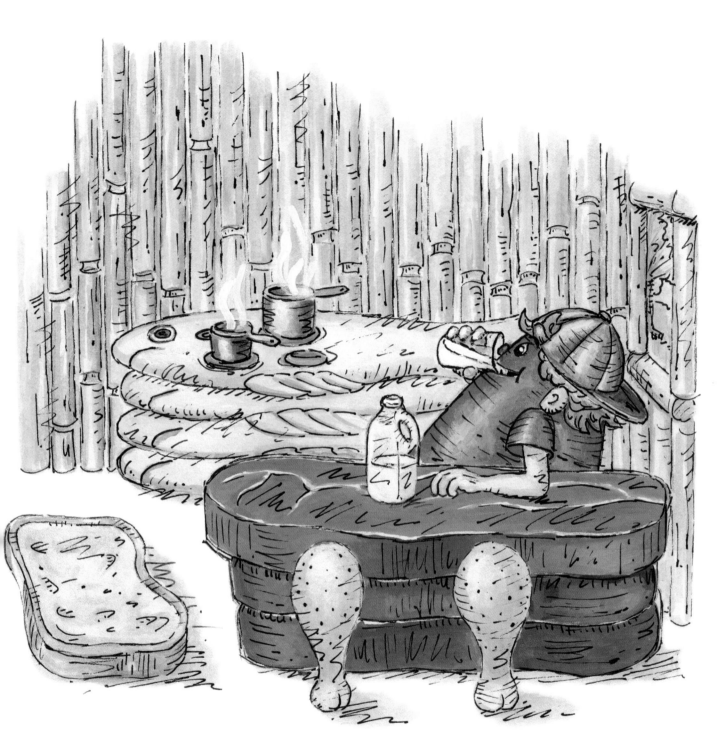

"I'll use chicken for stools, fish for a stove,
and a bar made of lean red meat.
Slices of whole wheat bread will serve
as comfy rugs under my feet."

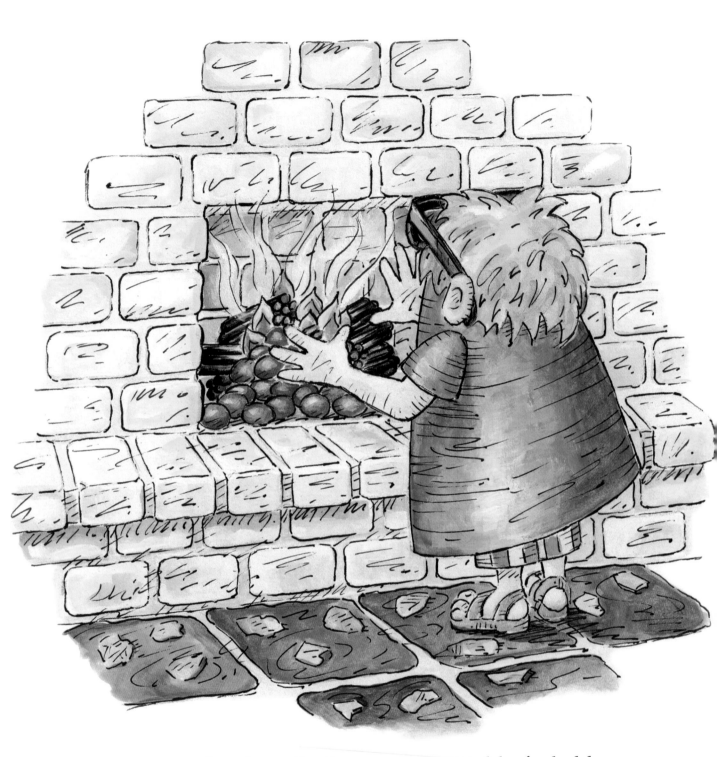

"For a fireplace that's cozy when cold winds blow, nothing's better than bubble gum bricks.
To keep me warm I choose oodles of red hots, and licorice is perfect for sticks!"

"I'll make my gutters from celery stalks.
They'll gather up water for sure.
I'll stick a spigot into each orange
to deliver juice fresh and pure!"

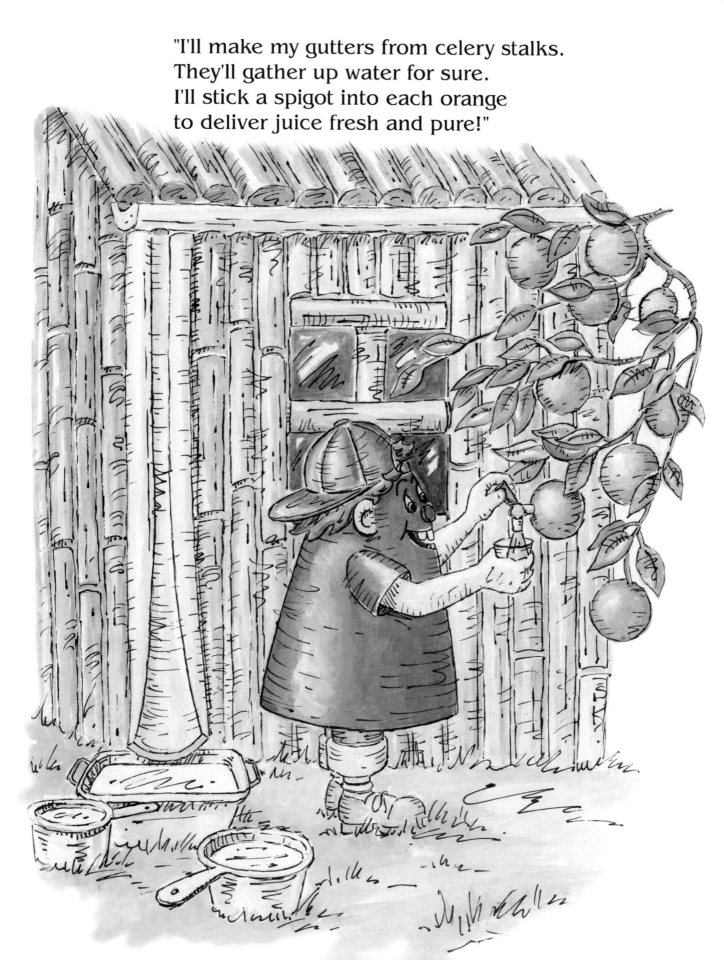

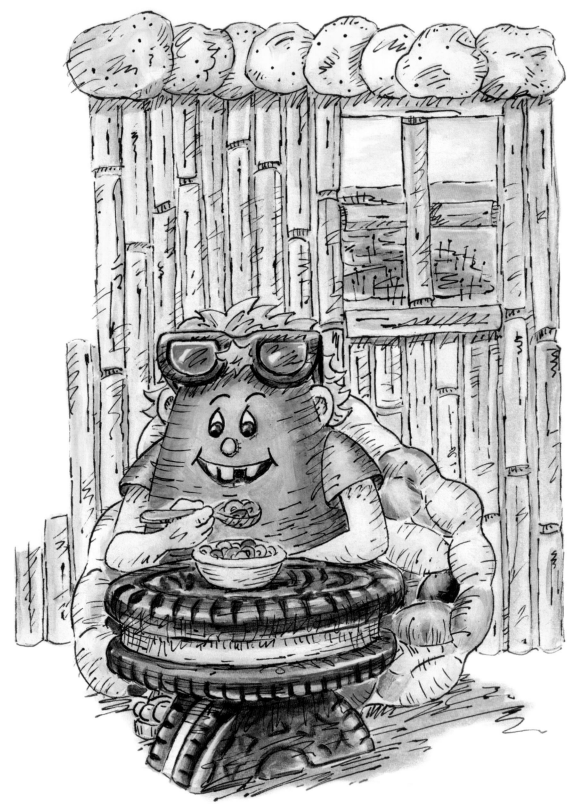

"A chocolate cookie filled with creme
is the table on which I eat.
And a jelly beanbag chair will surely
make a yummy seat!"

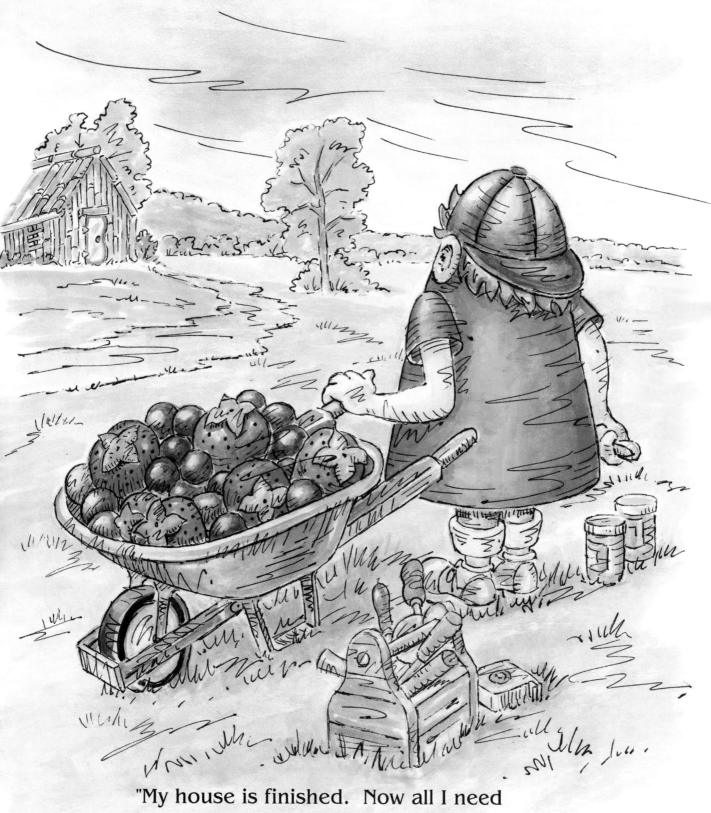

"My house is finished. Now all I need
is a strong, delicious fence.
Blueberries and strawberries should do the trick.
They're perfect! I'll spare no expense."

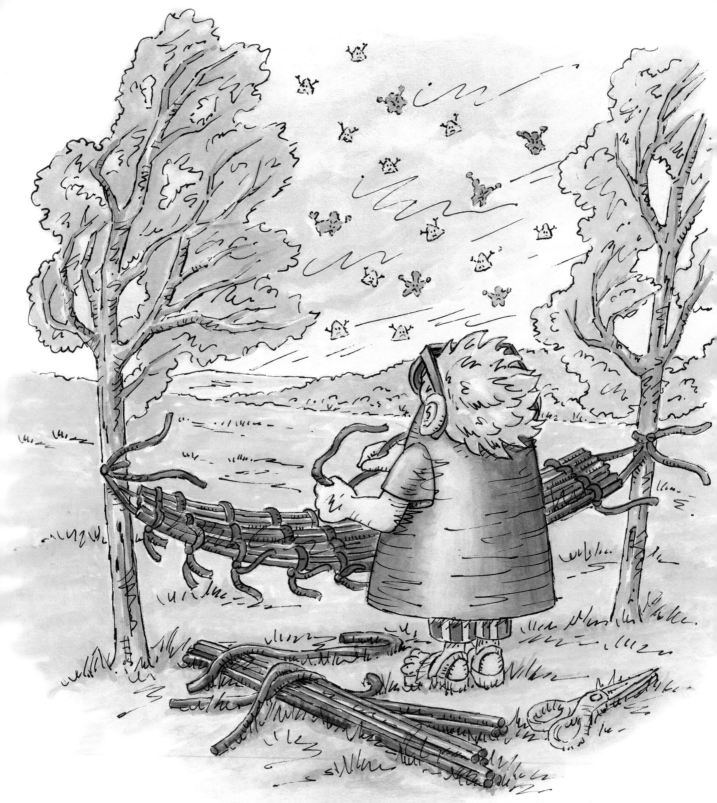

"Can't wait to relax in my hammock so sweet.
Oh, no . . . what's that in the sky?
Looks like a vicious whirlwind of germs,
and they're on the attack. Oh, my!"

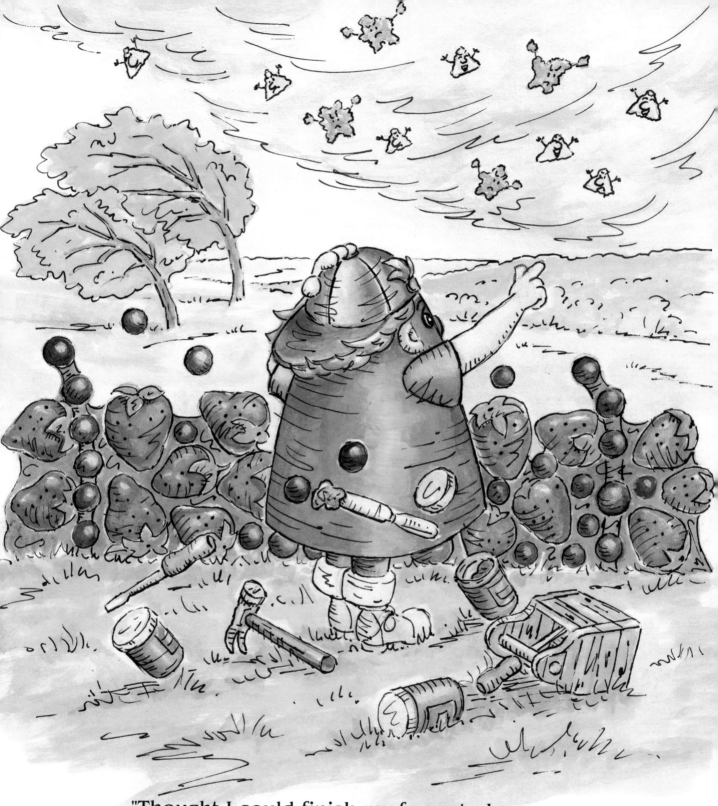

"Thought I could finish my fence today,
but the wind's really starting to blow!
The sky's turning dark. Are those germs in the air?
What happened? Where'd the sun go?"

"I'm scared of that ugly tornado.
It's filled with coughs and colds.
I better head for my 'Home Sweet Home'
and hope my roof won't fold!"

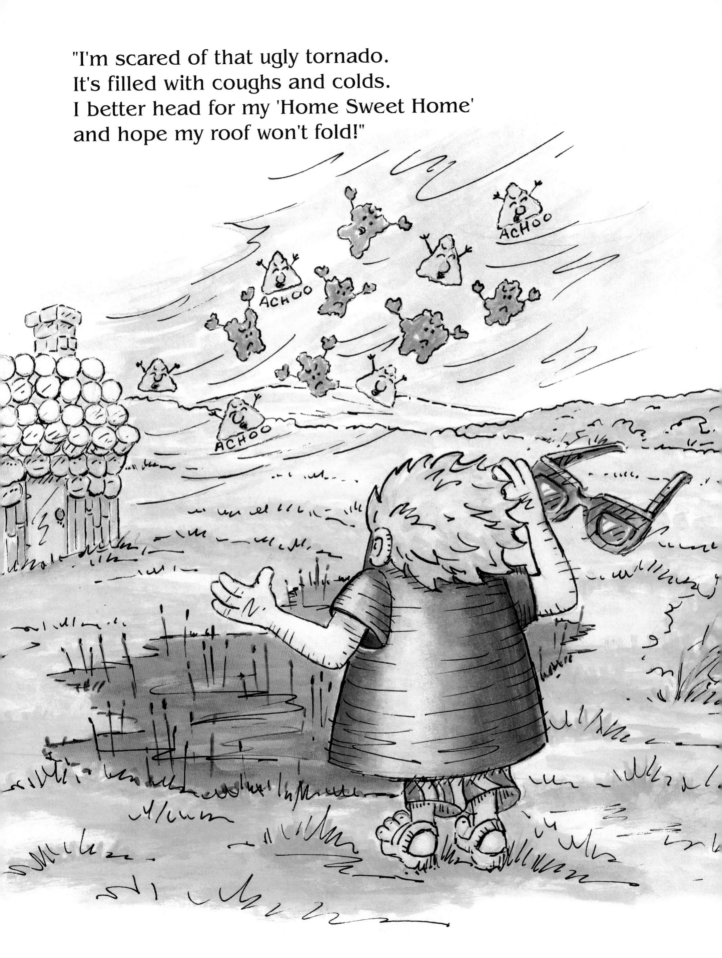

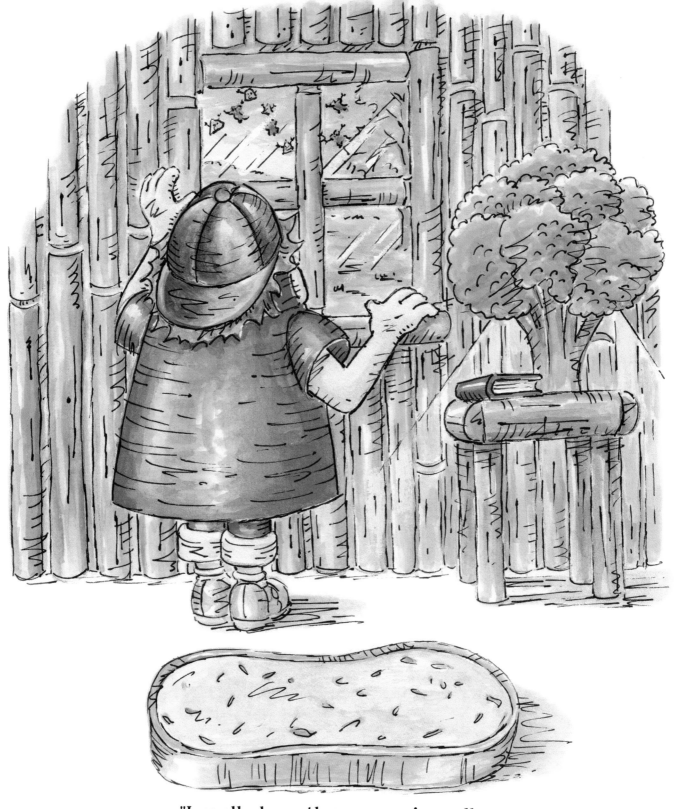

"I really love these veggie walls.
They keep me safe and dry.
That virus cannot get inside.
The storm will pass me by!"

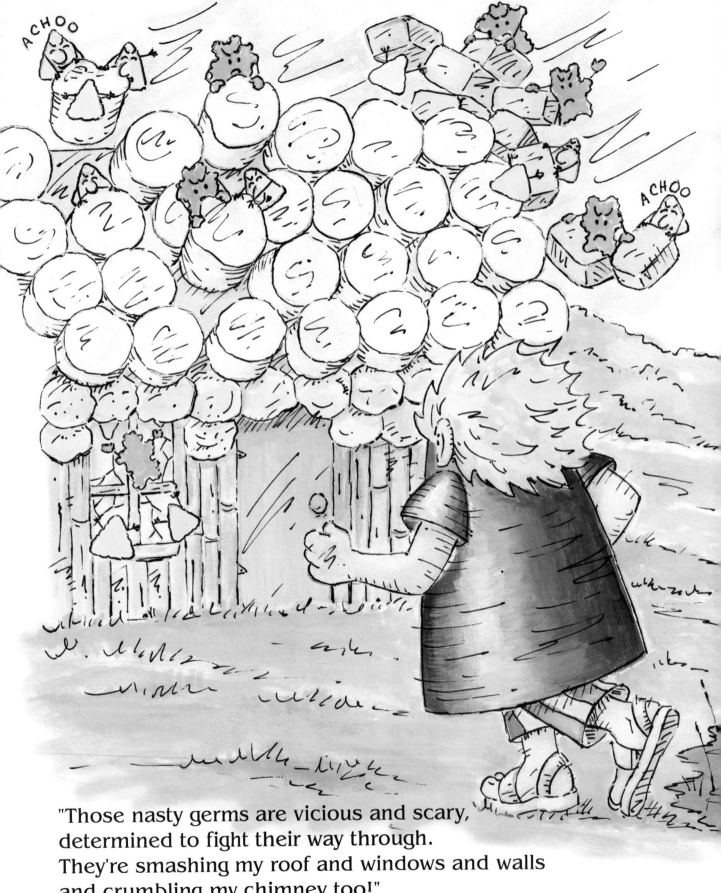

"Those nasty germs are vicious and scary,
determined to fight their way through.
They're smashing my roof and windows and walls
and crumbling my chimney too!"

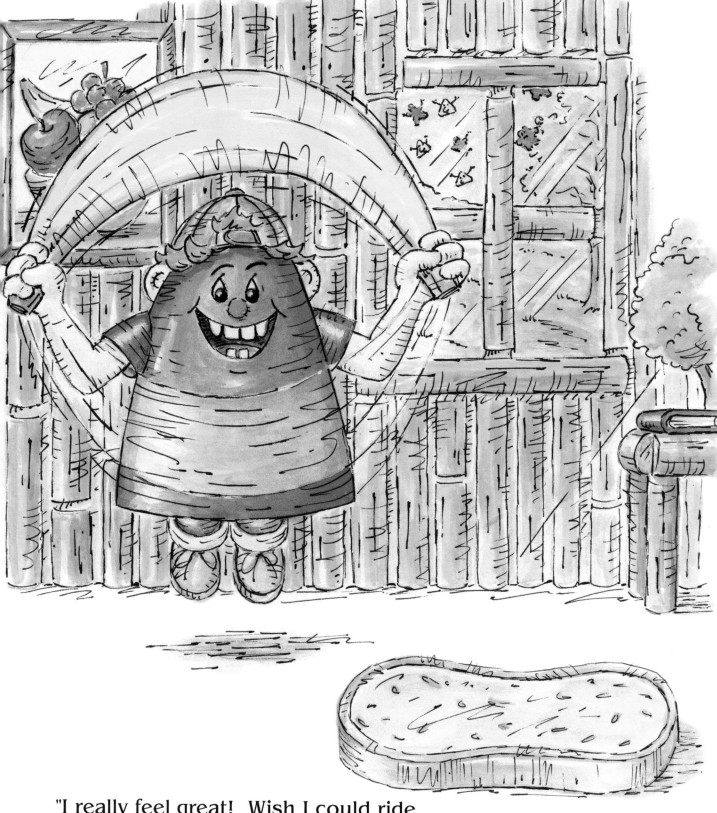

"I really feel great! Wish I could ride
my bike for exercise.
But because of the storm pounding my walls,
I'll have to work out inside."

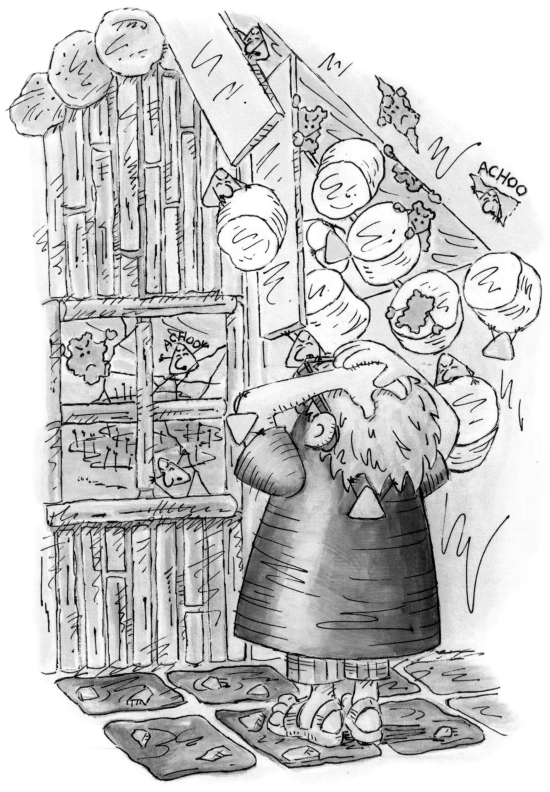

"My marshmallow roof is crashing down!
It wasn't tough and thick.
Germs broke through—made a brutal attack.
Now I'm dizzy and sick!"

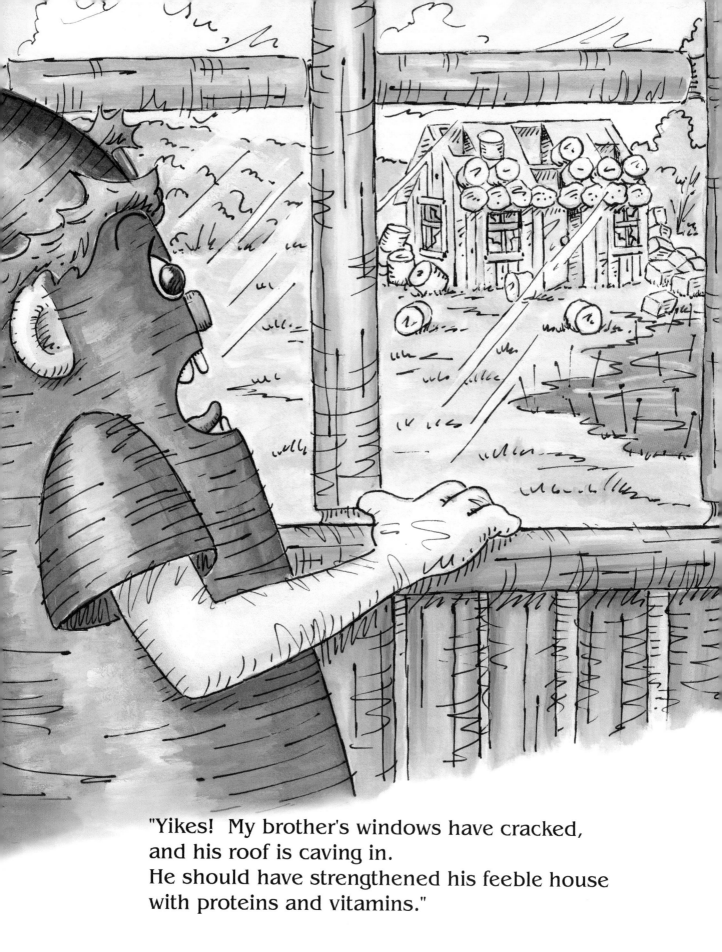

"Yikes! My brother's windows have cracked,
and his roof is caving in.
He should have strengthened his feeble house
with proteins and vitamins."

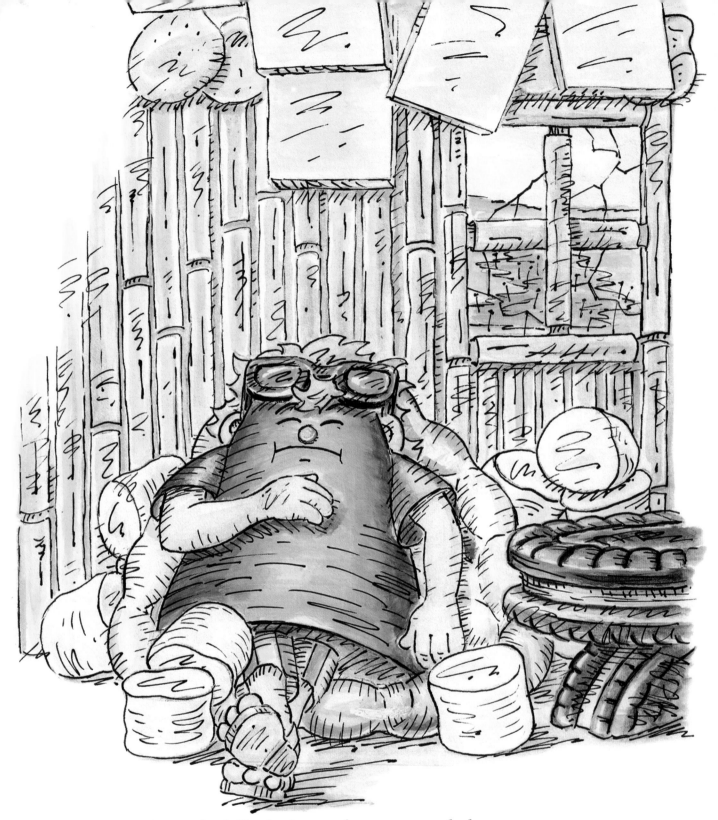

"I'm glad that storm is over and done.
I should make repairs.
But I feel so wobbly and weak,
think I'll snooze in my beanbag chair."

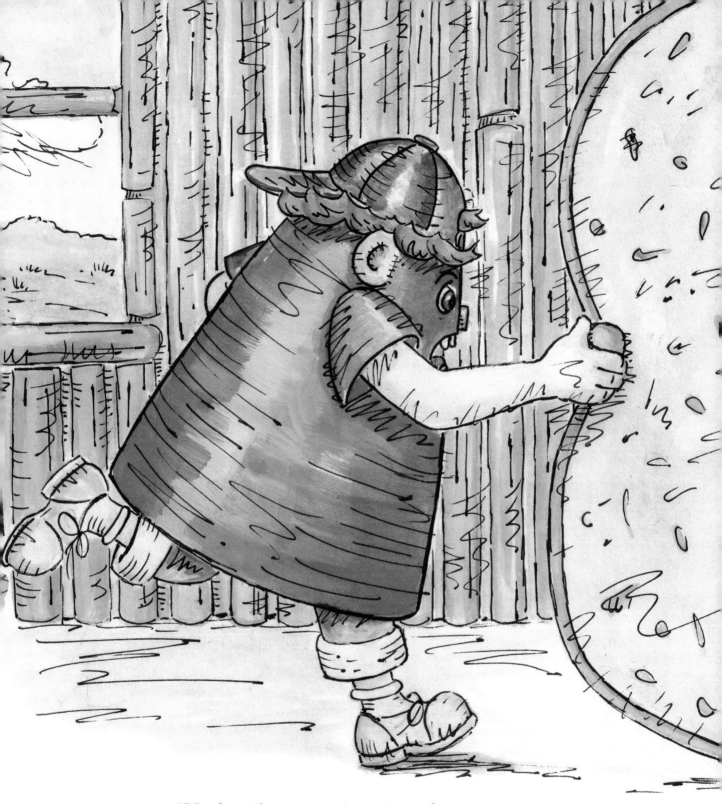

"My brother needs a lot of help.
My fence will have to wait.
His house is toppling to the ground.
I'll hurry. I can't be late!"

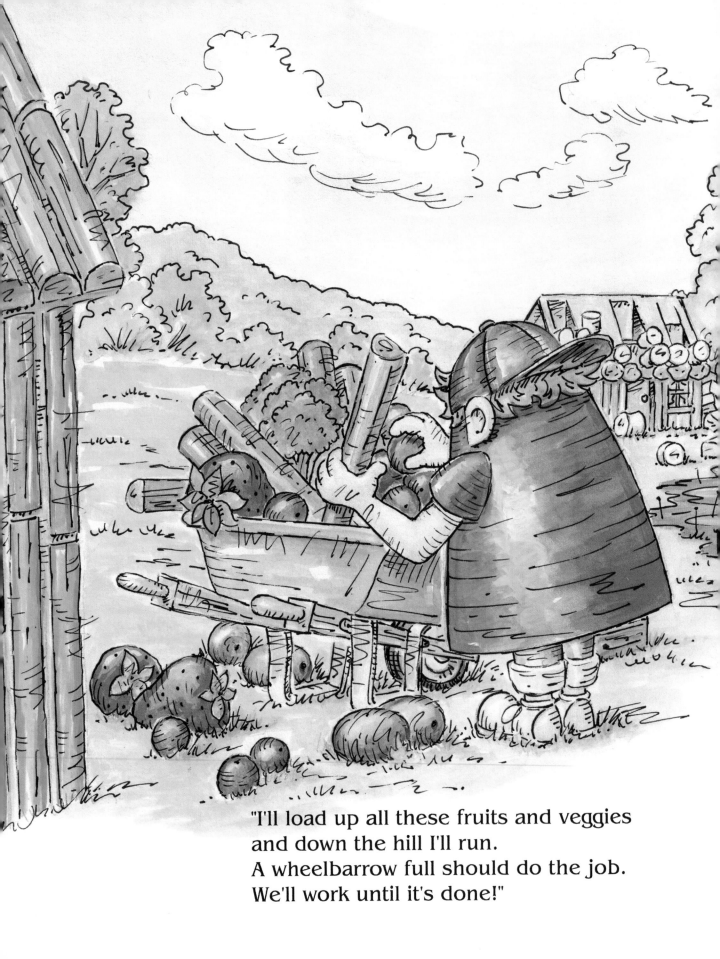

"I'll load up all these fruits and veggies
and down the hill I'll run.
A wheelbarrow full should do the job.
We'll work until it's done!"

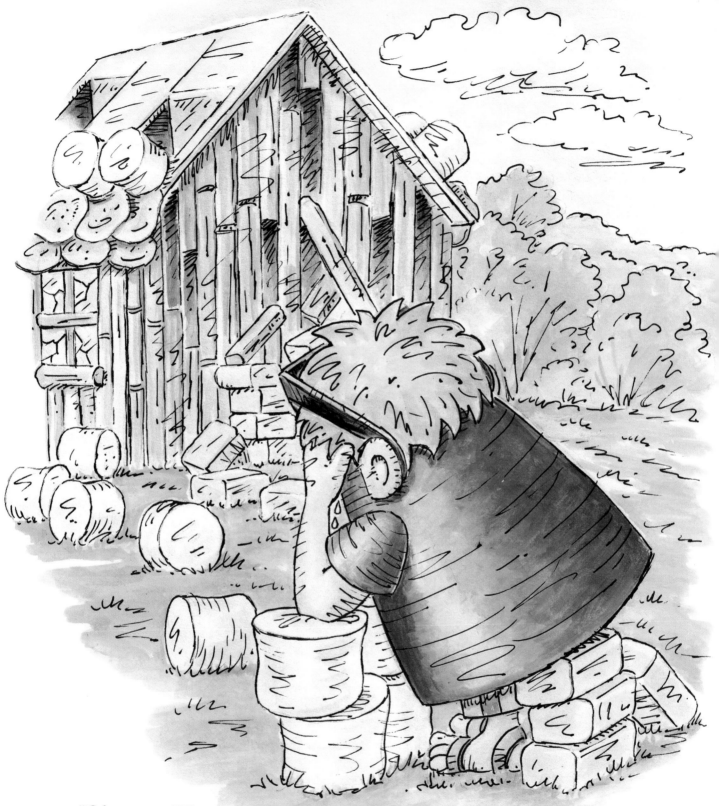

"Oh, no. What a mess I've made of my home!
I've never been so blue.
My windows broke, the chimney fell,
and my poor roof caved in too!"

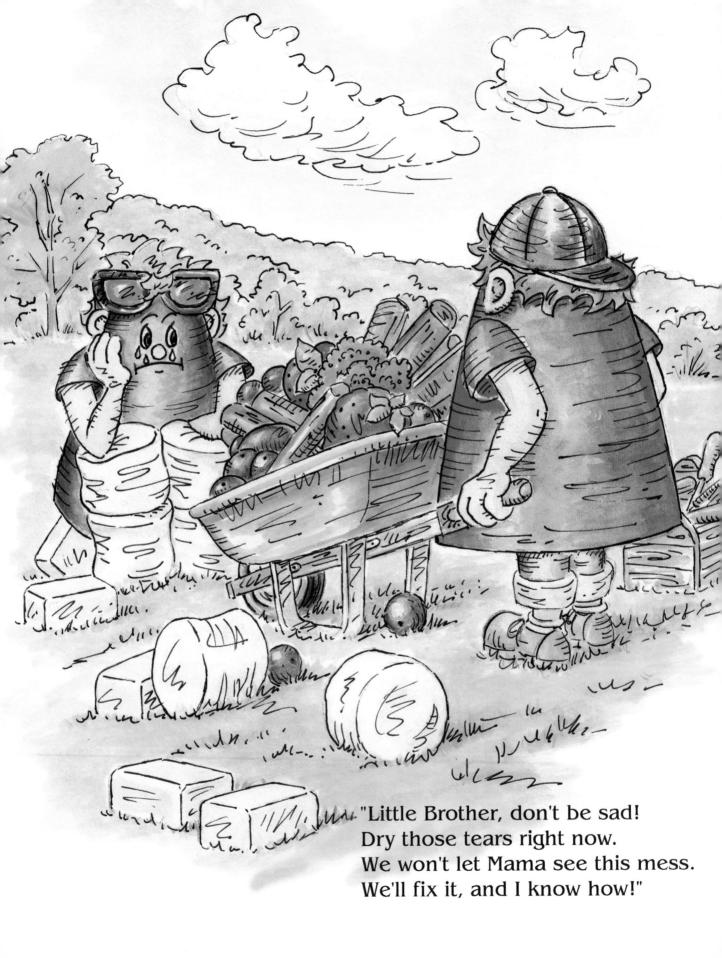

"Little Brother, don't be sad!
Dry those tears right now.
We won't let Mama see this mess.
We'll fix it, and I know how!"

"I came to help since I see why
you're in this crazy funk.
Your house did not protect you well
'cause it's made of nothing but junk!"

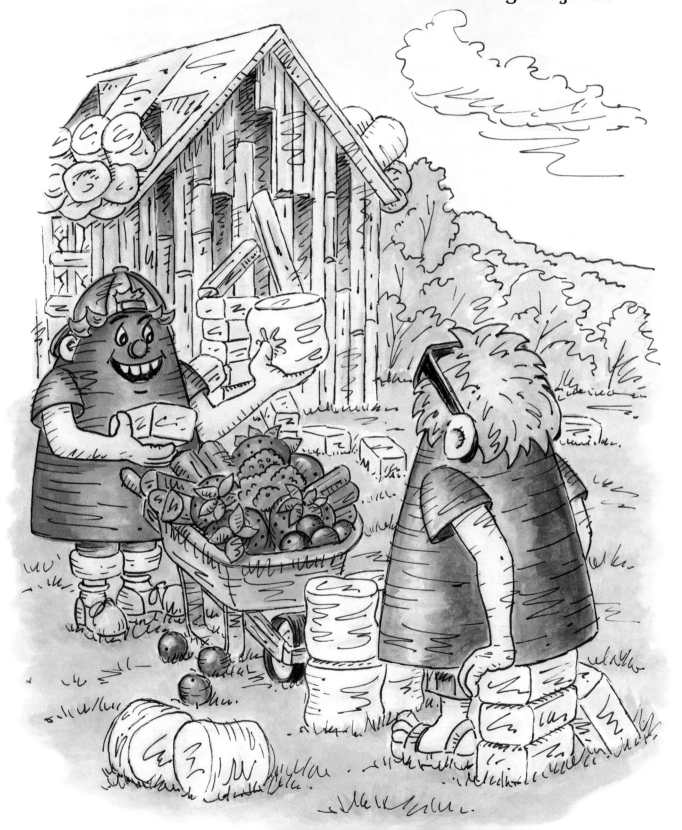

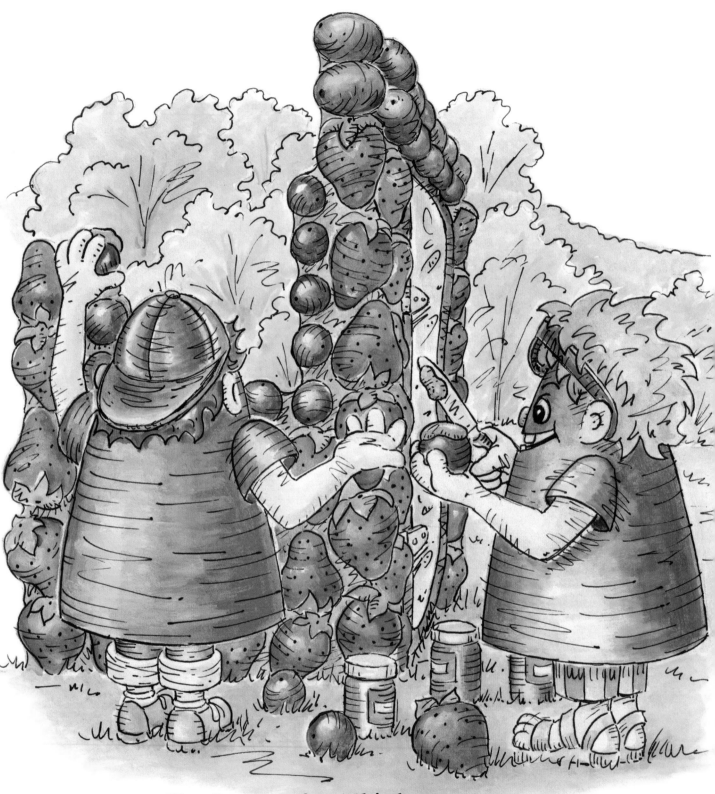

"Don't worry about this humongous mess.
Your place will soon look great.
For when you build with healthy foods,
you'll learn it's NEVER too late!"

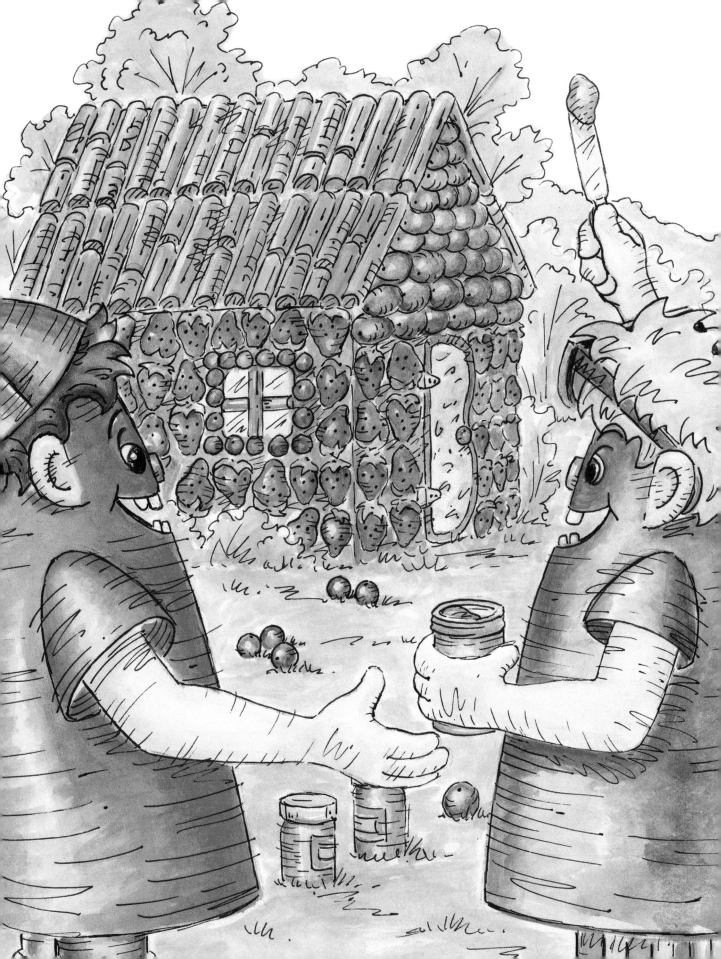

Made in the USA
Charleston, SC
03 May 2013